THE MODERN CAVEMAN
A GUIDE TO A HEALTHIER YOU THROUGH A PALEO DIET, EXERCISE, AND ALTERNATIVE MEDICINE
AF810830
DR. CARL BAMLET D.C., C.N.S.

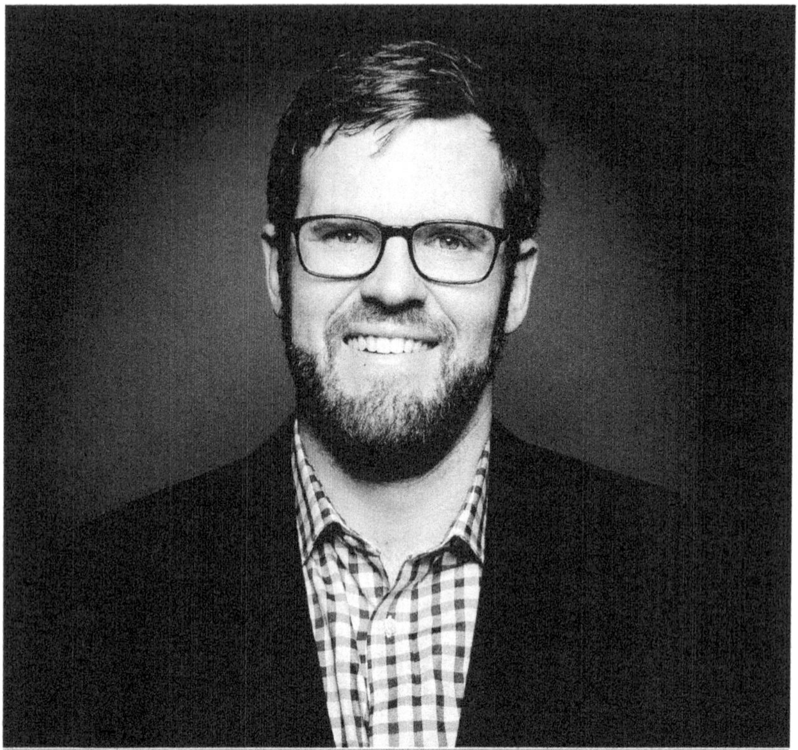

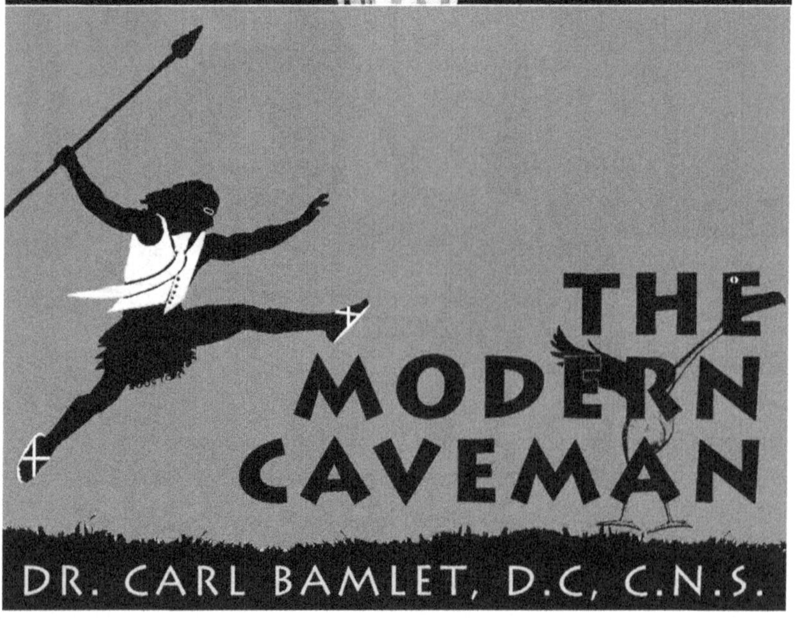
THE
MODERN
CAVEMAN
DR. CARL BAMLET, D.C, C.N.S.

The Modern Caveman

A Guide to a Healthier You Through a Paleo Diet, Exercise, and Alternative Medicine

Dr. Carl Bamlet D.C., C.N.S.

ISBN: 978-1-944878-07-8

Published by JETLAUNCH
www.jetlaunch.net

Be the change you want to see in the world.

Mahatma Ghandi

TABLE OF CONTENTS

Meet the Author

For such a young man, Dr. Bamlet has attained an admirable amount of wisdom—wisdom that comes from first-hand experience—and his interest in nutrition stems back many years. With a history and background in sports and athletic pursuits, his passion for chiropractic and alternative medicine began.

He recollects an event that sparked his desire to pursue his career in medicine when he sustained a wrestling injury to his neck and shoulder. Upon consulting an M.D., he was told he had a pinched nerve. He was prescribed painkillers and muscle relaxants and was told to stand down from wrestling for two weeks. For Carl, this didn't seem like a great option, so he visited a chiropractor who adjusted his neck and released some trigger points. This enabled Carl to return to wrestling practice that same day. The almost instantaneous results proved just how incredible chiropractic could be.

While Carl was studying at college a few years later, he was diagnosed with brain cancer. The endless array of specialist consults and six months of cancer treatments helped Carl come to the realisation that the medical profession doesn't understand what causes a majority of our chronic health challenges. Through his direct and relentless questioning and observations, he found that whilst they understood what was happening in the body physically and had discovered how to treat the related symptoms, they did not know the causes, or often, how best to prevent them. The place for this traditional medicine is very relevant for emergency treatment, some cancers, and various other conditions, but through his own illness and rehabilitation, he discovered that the way to become healthy and maintain that was for it to become his lifestyle. The spark had ignited into a real passion for natural medicine.

After finishing his undergraduate degree, Dr. Bamlet attended chiropractic school, and while there, sought to also further his education in nutrition. Alongside his full time chiropractic studies, he attended two weekend seminars per month and began reading and listening to every resource available, through numerous books, CDs and DVDs. He soon began the process of taking in all of the information available, and with further research, was able to eliminate some and focus on what he believed to be the most useful. His studies continued, and upon graduation from chiropractic school, he went on to gain a certificate in Chiropractic Acupuncture and qualified as a Certified Nutrition Specialist.

Once qualified, and with a host of relevant certificates and degrees to his name, Dr. Bamlet accepted an exciting role in New Zealand and knew this would be a fantastic opportunity to master his craft. Dr. Bamlet is now licensed to practice in two countries and the opportunities to hone his career and pass on his knowledge and passion for health, wellness, and nutrition continue to present themselves.

By utilising his expertise and skills, he provides a transparent approach to health, medicine, and treatments to assist you in accessing the best information. This enables you to make informed choices on your most important asset: your health and well-being.

If you would like to know more about Dr. Carl, check out these links.

www.plainsfm.co.nz
(Dr. Carl Bamlet: The Modern Caveman radio show)

www.epicmentors.co.nz/magazine/Issue 45

www.spectatornews.com/student-life/2007/11/08/grappling-with-cancer

www.goo.gl/0S90q1

Acknowledgments

I would like to thank the following:

Dr. John O'Malley

Dr. Laura Pirkl

Gene Bamlet

Mary Bamlet

Chris O'Byrne and JETLAUNCH Publishing

INTRODUCTION

Although the title of this book may have piqued your interest, it is impossible to determine whether or not cavemen had cancer. However, it's highly likely that cavemen died from sustaining traumatic injuries from battle wounds, poisonous animals, or other significant events.

The book's title is meant to provoke thought around eating right, exercising, and the significant role this plays in the development of cancer and degenerative disease. These are two concerns that are becoming increasingly important issues in Western civilization. Although we cannot categorically say that cavemen didn't have cancer, we can definitively say that cave children 20,000 years ago didn't suffer the escalating rates of childhood cancer, orthopedic surgeries, diabetes, and obesity. Children even three generations ago didn't have these conditions at the levels they do now. If you read this book from an emotional connection to your food and beliefs instead of with a constructive and open viewpoint, your benefits may be minimal.

How often has this scenario happened to you or a loved one?

Dr: "There's nothing wrong with you."

You: "What do you mean? Then why am I having these headaches? Why do I feel so fatigued?"

Dr: "The bloodwork and MRI came back negative; there's nothing wrong with you. This is part of getting older." Or "The bloodwork and MRI came back negative; there's nothing wrong with you. We want you to see this psychiatrist." Or the worst case. "The bloodwork and MRI came back negative; take these pills."

Speaking from personal experience and numerous patient recollections, this is an all-too-common occurrence, and even once is unacceptable. You pay for a consultation because something feels wrong and you want an answer. Even if the answer is, "I don't know what's wrong," it's still an appropriate response—not ideal, but acceptable—and you respect the doctor for admitting they don't know. In this instance, you leave wondering who can help, and you are motivated to seek alternative treatment elsewhere instead of being embarrassed and or depressed.

In the coming chapters, you will learn the benefits and weaknesses of Western and Eastern medicines, the Paleolithic diet, what types of practitioners you should look for locally to avoid the scenario mentioned above, along with many other health concerns.

Section 1

Western Medicine

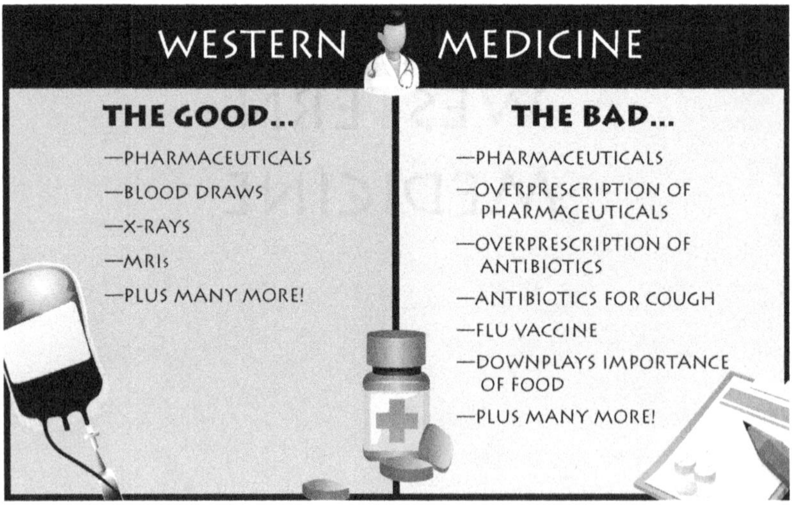
WESTERN MEDICINE
THE GOOD...
—PHARMACEUTICALS
—BLOOD DRAWS
—X-RAYS
—MRIs
—PLUS MANY MORE!
THE BAD...
—PHARMACEUTICALS
—OVERPRESCRIPTION OF PHARMACEUTICALS
—OVERPRESCRIPTION OF ANTIBIOTICS
—ANTIBIOTICS FOR COUGH
—FLU VACCINE
—DOWNPLAYS IMPORTANCE OF FOOD
—PLUS MANY MORE!

CHAPTER 1

DEFINING WESTERN/MODERN MEDICINE

What is meant by Western or modern medicine? The image that most of us have when we talk about Western medicine is of diagnoses that match an array of symptoms to a known paradigm of diseases and dysfunctions by utilizing lab tests, advanced imaging (MRI, X-ray), and genetics. If science can't visualize or measure it, then it must not exist—or it is left unconsidered, which is the same as not existing.

In order to fully understand the definition given above, we need to have a clear understanding of what a disease is. Can you define disease? Look in the dictionary for a clear definition. Still can't find a clear definition? Type 2 diabetes and obesity are considered diseases, as is tuberculosis, and AIDS, to name a few. Until 1974, homosexuality was classified as a disease. This illustrates just how much confusion exists around defining "disease." But we have to be able to define health, right?

The World Health Organization has made a valiant attempt at defining health as, "A state of complete physical, mental, and social well-being, not merely the absence of disease or infirmity." This attempt to define health has received criticism for not being realistic or being too wildly utopian. After all, how dare we aim to be happy and healthy?

Practitioners of Western medicine are M.D.s, D.O.s, D.P.M.s, D.C.s (to some extent), nurse practitioners, nutritionists, dieticians, and most practitioners you find in a hospital setting. Within each of these fields are dramatically varying viewpoints on many topics. For example, certain M.D.s are opposed to the use of pharmaceuticals and some D.C.s are in favor of pharmaceuticals.

You will find this paper in EMBO which discusses what a disease is to be an excellent reference. http://bit.ly/21cE0zL

Chapter 2

Strengths of Western Medicine

Western medicine has many advantages over its Eastern counterparts in most aspects of disease management. I will endeavour to outline throughout this book the differences between a disease and lifestyle-created ailments that as a society we call "disease."

Surgery

You would want your essential surgeries performed by the most specialized doctor, using the most sophisticated imaging and tools. In 1000 A.D., a surgeon probably didn't have a high survival rate. Obviously, the overzealous recommendation for surgeries, along with an overwhelming majority of the population that is unwilling to take accountability for their own health, is a different topic.

Understanding of anatomy, physiology, histology and pathology

The modern understanding of physiology, histology, and pathology is incredible. The amazing detail with which we can image anatomy and measure physiological and pathological function is very beneficial in monitoring the disease process. It gives us an understanding of what is happening, but it doesn't address why it is happening. This knowledge is usually obtained by acquiring a bachelor's degree in human biology. Continued studies progress knowledge in your field while solidifying the basic sciences.

Anaesthetics

Anaesthetics have helped transform surgery into a much more pleasant and successful process. Without such drugs, survival rates would drop dramatically because the patient would be awake and in agonizing pain, resulting in the surgeon's inability to perform a thorough procedure, or the patient going into shock and dying.

Treating red flags

Red flags are symptoms that warn you of a more serious underlying condition (e.g. sudden onset of intense left arm and neck pain often indicate myocardial infarction). Red flags such as unintentional rapid weight loss, loss of consciousness, plus several more, often indicate a more serious underlying condition and are often differentially diagnosed by your M.D. with an array of expensive equipment provided by the hospital. This is an amazing aspect of Western medicine and technology.

Pain killers

Pain killers are indispensable when they are absolutely needed, and can be found in many forms. Some are addictive, some are not, some are stronger than others, but when we wake from a surgery after we were hit by a runaway car, we are very grateful they exist. Our society's over-dependence on them is not the fault of the pain killers or the doctors who prescribe them.

Pharmaceuticals for genetic disorders along with diagnosis to understand what's happening

When a genetic mutation or alteration occurs, producing an extra chromosome, or when your body lacks the ability to create blood clotting factors, for example, Western medicine can identify what happened and what can be done. Without drugs for these purposes, our loved ones life expectancy could dramatically decrease.

Taking a clotting factor made in a lab is about the only way to stop a haemophiliac from bleeding endlessly. Without drugs for these purposes, life expectancy is dramatically decreased.

CHAPTER 3

WEAKNESSES OF WESTERN MEDICINE

Health

No one goes to their medical doctor because they are healthy and want to maintain their health. Your annual check-up is to investigate for the first signs of disease. The information and tools that the medical community uses are meant to help diagnose and treat disease. This is very important but has little significance in staying healthy.

No disease ever resulted from the lack of a pharmaceutical, a chemical made in a lab by humans that does not exist in the natural world. All a pharmaceutical does is hide the symptoms and often creates new ones. The same goes for removing organs and other useful body parts. Removing your gallbladder may temporarily relieve you of the pain created from your bad habits, but that pain was in fact an early warning sign. It's an indication of future issues arising from an unhealthy lifestyle such as consuming copious amounts of coffee and deep-fried foods.

Propensity towards surgeries

There is still a large element of risk through complications of surgical procedures, even with modern technology. The staggering numbers of surgeries performed are due to the medical profession's apparent opinion that surgery should be viewed as a first option in treatment. The predominant way of thinking in the general public is that surgery is an easy option and that modern procedures guarantee safety, therefore producing a reluctance to change our lifestyle and habits because it's perceived as too difficult. Our reluctance to change our habits also contributes to the high rates of surgery, as the popular thought is that the easy way (surgery) is safe and the hard way (changing habits and lifestyle) isn't worth it.

"Genetic predisposition"

Your genes are not your destiny. Through the work done on the human genome project, we know that epigenetics play a much more important role than our genes.

Epigenetics address the environmental and lifestyle factors we are exposed to that affects how our genes express themselves. This means that beer, burger, and fries followed by sitting on the couch day after day will turn on the bad genes. However, a steak, seasonal vegetables, and fruit salad, followed by a walk, run, or other physical activity, will turn on the good genes.

The main reason pharmaceutical companies and mainstream medicine aren't informing us about epigenetics is that it doesn't make money for them. You can't sell a pill that is a substitute for exercise and good food, but you can sell a pill for bad genes you can't do anything about.

For more information on this topic I recommend the following TED talk by Dean Ornish, a clinical professor at UCSF and founder of the Preventive Medicine Research Institute. http://bit.ly/1qhUJnv

We have forgotten the importance of food

The importance of nutrition is largely left unmentioned by the medical community, and through this neglect, it lacks importance in their eyes. Most medical doctors feel diet is not even a factor in the disease process. Even for conditions such as Type 2 diabetes, gout, and high cholesterol (some forms of high cholesterol are due to Familial hypercholesterolemia, a genetic variant), the medical establishment's stance is that diet and lifestyle play little or no part in the disease, and pills or surgery are the best or only answer.

Even when the medical establishment recommends supplements, they are often sourced from ingredients processed in a lab using heat, intense pressure, or chemicals. This process alters the energetic configuration, and alters how our body recognizes and utilizes it. Rarely, if ever, are over-the-counter supplements tested for efficacy (nutrients working to create a desired effect).

Only civilization that hasn't accepted some form of energetic outline to the body

In Western medicine, we know that the body creates a resting membrane potential of approximately -65 to -75 mV using the sodium potassium pump, in part, to achieve this. This is a basic principle that is driven home early in your human biology curriculum. I realize this doesn't directly correlate to classical electrical currents that humans have measured, and fully understand, but let's examine a little about what we know and postulate about what we don't. A principal of classical electromagnetism is Ampere's law. This law states that an electrical current will have an electromagnetic field proportional to its strength.

In Western medicine a device called a magnetocardiogram (MCG) can be used to measure the heart's magnetic field. It's possible this bit of information would have been outside your realm of believability just a few seconds ago and the MCG is still pretty basic, in the realm of what is possible. What is so special about the heart? Why is it the only organ with a biomagnetic field? These are valid questions, and the answer I will offer is this:

All the organs are special, and they all possess some form of a biomagnetic field. That principle is what many other civilizations have known for thousands of years.

The Hindus have passed down their energetic representation to the body through the 7-chakra system which many of us would recognize. Tibetan's have a 6-chakra system, the Mayan had a 7-chakra system, the Cherokee had a 7-chakra system, and the Incas had their own energy system. The Jewish have the ancient Kabbalah. Perhaps the most recognizable of all is the acupuncture 12-meridian system. This is not all of the energy representations that have existed in the world, and if you would like to learn more, I highly recommend *The Subtle Body* by Cyndi Dale.

I argue that just because humankind isn't smart enough to measure and quantify an energy system, that this in no way means an energy system does not exist. It only means we aren't smart enough yet. My recommendation to you is try out the different forms using several different practitioners until you find the right one. If Ayurveda is not for you, then try acupuncture. If acupuncture doesn't sit well, try homeopathy. If homeopathy doesn't feel right, try reiki. If reiki is not working for you, try the next option, until you find the right fit for you. I've personally experienced acupuncture, and that resonates with me. Ayurveda is another aspect that interests me, and I plan on looking into it in the future.

Still practice germ theory

Germs—bacteria and viruses—are always around us. Bacteria and viruses are not what make us sick, otherwise we would constantly be sick. Bacteria and viruses are opportunistic, which means they succeed in infecting us only when we are in a weakened state. When our immune systems are suppressed by sugar, stress, lack of sleep, open wounds, and many other causes, then germs can infect us. There are viruses and germs like the HIV virus, and treponema pallidum (syphilis) that our immune system can't fight on its own, but they have to get into the body first.

Yet we are prescribed antibiotics for every condition, from acne to earaches (earaches are treated with antibiotics, in case the pain may be from an ear infection). We vaccinate everyone for common viruses like influenza to chicken pox. You may think I am opposed to all vaccines and antibiotics, but I am not. What I am opposed to is the continual overuse of these crutches in improper situations largely for financial gain.

Study of animal populations has led us to hypothesize that these bacteria and viruses exist to kill off the weakest of the species and to prevent overpopulation, thus ensuring survival of the fittest. But, as we use more antibiotics and vaccines, we see nature changing to once again eliminate the weakest. Methicillin-resistant Staphylococcus aureus (MRSA) is the most obvious example of this. We should not blame the medical practitioners for recommending this solution, as they often have pressure applied by the patient to prescribe these solutions. The fault lies in the system—but how can we change it?

The answer is in this book.

Direct to consumer marketing

Direct-to-consumer marketing is the epitome of what is wrong with our healthcare system. We have the most corrupt sector of medicine, with pharmaceutical companies brainwashing the general public with their marketing, resulting in them applying pressure on their medical practitioner to get the latest drug when they usually don't need it. The general public has little or no knowledge of biochemistry, physiology, pharmacology, or medicine, yet it is to them that we directly market the most dangerous aspect of healthcare for profits.

The U.S. is a giant science experiment on what side effects like mass drugging (among other co-factors like poor diet and lack of exercise) will have on the health of a society. The experiment is failing.

In 2003, the U.S. consumed 45% of all pharmaceuticals globally. (http://apps.who.int/medicinedocs/en/d/Js6160e/6.html) In 2000, the U.S. was ranked 38th by the WHO in terms of health. The U.S. spends the most on healthcare and pharmaceuticals in the world and yet only ranks 38th in health. Clearly, something isn't working.

SECTION 2

EASTERN/TRADITIONAL MEDICINE

CHAPTER 4

DEFINING EASTERN/TRADITIONAL MEDICINE

What is meant by Eastern/traditional medicine? The image that most have when we talk about Eastern medicine is of energy medicine, acupuncture meridians, medicine men, herbal preparations, or supplements. Often, the Westernized world thinks of these things as being weird, unusual, or crazy, which are all ways to express that we are scared to think that they might possibly be correct. We are scared because it's so far outside of our paradigm of possibility, that if this weird stuff can be true, what other unshakable truths become less definite? If cancer, diabetes, Parkinsons, etc. aren't just bad luck (bad genes, same thing as bad luck), but in fact are created by our environment's interactions with our genes (epigenetics), what other scary things might be true? This realization forces most of us to close off and not pose any further questions.

What Eastern medicine stands for is finding out what is affecting the body negatively and removing that insulting factor, whether it be an energetic, emotional, nutritional, or structural disturbance. Then, a treatment takes place to remove insulting factors, replace essential nutrients, or realign the structural integrity of the body.

Practitioners of Eastern/traditional medicine would be D.C.s (to some extent), acupuncturists, naturopaths, massage therapists, Ayurvedic medicine practitioners, herbalists, and many more.

CHAPTER 5

STRENGTHS OF EASTERN MEDICINE

Eastern medicine has many advantages over its Western counterparts in most aspects of health and disease prevention.

Energetic body

Traditional Chinese medicine has learned an incredible amount about the energetic body over the past 6,000 years. Ayurvedic medicine has an equally impressive understanding of the energetic body, which has been formed over the same amount of time.

Ampere's Law states, "The magnetic field in space around an electric current is proportional to the electric current which serves as its source, just as the electric field in space is proportional to the charge, which serves as its source." While Amperes Law is usually applied regarding traditional electrical currents, it can also be argued that it applies to bioelectrical currents as well.Magnetocardiograms (MCG) measure the heart's electromagnetic field using sensitive devices known as SQUIDS (superconducting quantum interference device). Western medical technology is beginning to measure what Eastern medicine has known for thousands of years, but the principles behind these even existing still isn't widely accepted in Western medicine. The heart is the most well-known of our organs, but every organ has its own magnetic field to measure.

Skeletal health

Chiropractic is far newer (formed in 1895) than both Ayurveda and acupuncture, but the principles of chiropractic, correcting bony structure misalignments which are causing pain and weakness, have been around since before Hippocrates. Yes, Hippocrates performed bony manipulations. Chiropractic calls the energetic aspect of the body innate intelligence.

Nutrition

Eastern medicine values the energetics of food in making a nutritional supplement. If you heat the compound, you change the energetic composition of it. If you use chemical reagents to extract parts of the food, you also change the structure. Even putting the compound under intense pressure will change the energetic configuration. What is the difference between coal and diamonds? It is intense pressure and heat that changes coal into diamonds.

These chemistry facts are the absolute basics of nutrition that need to be understood. When all these factors are followed correctly, in the creation of a nutritional supplement, you still have to deal with something called biochemical individuality. Biochemical individuality simply means you are an individual, and your metabolic process will be slightly different than the next person.

Biochemical individuality exists because we all come from different parts of the world with our own locally available foods, which our bodies have learned to process. Bananas and coconuts wouldn't have been available in Norway or Minnesota 50,000 years ago, and likewise, corn and wheat wouldn't have been sourced in New Zealand or Fiji. Biochemical individuality is the reason why two people can take the same supplement and it may work for one and not the other. In Eastern medicine, muscle testing is a heuristic process, often used to identify what supplement, food, or treatment is right for you.

You're in control of your health

All these forms of medicine stress that you are in control of your own health. Your diet, exercise regime, state of mind, and mechanisms for coping with stress and lifestyle will determine how healthy you are. If slight imbalances occur, a natural health practitioner can assess this and recommend the correct nutrition, adjust the right bones, acupuncture the right points, identify food intolerances, or deliver some other form of natural intervention. Through identifying and altering these health challenges before they become disease, you will take control of your health. The common theme among most alternative medicine practitioners is that they claim to help an energetic aspect of the body along with a chemical or structural aspect.

Case study

A good example of how the energetic body can affect the structural body is scarring. In acupuncture, it's believed that scars can prevent or inhibit the flow of Qi (energy). Scars can be treated using acupuncture needles, castor oil packs, or mud packing, among other ways.

With the use of chiropractic and nutrition, I was able to significantly help one patient with most of his complaints, except for his left shoulder. His shoulder would be corrected for a week, and then, when the wind was strong, his shoulder would hurt again. This doesn't correlate with any chiropractic or nutrition thought process, but it does resonate in acupuncture.

During a visit where I was learning about the wind's ability to cause the issue with the shoulder, I started to investigate this patient for scars. I found that an old scar on his right knee, caused by a serious car accident, was the source of the shoulder pain. The surgeon had done an excellent job, as he is able to walk marvellously. Several acupuncture treatments and castor oil packs later, his pain was gone and has stayed away. The moral of this story, besides the obvious, is that if your doctor, regardless of the initials after their name, doesn't listen to your observations and offer possible solutions, find one that does.

Chapter 6

Weaknesses of Eastern Medicine

Eastern medicine is not without its downsides.

Emergency situations

Eastern medicine does not handle emergency situations well, at all. If you're shot, stabbed, hit by a car, having a heart attack, having a stroke, or have broken a bone that it is protruding through the skin, you'd be wise go to a hospital because alternative medicine is limited as to what it can help. Adjustments, acupuncture, meditation, yoga, and any other natural treatment can do absolutely nothing for internal bleeding and compound fractures and other life-threatening injuries.

Patient motivation

Another limitation of Eastern medicine is that the patient needs some motivation to be healthy. Diet and exercise are vital to being healthy, and as powerful as chiropractic adjustments, acupuncture, massage, and nutritional supplements are, they cannot overcome a terrible diet and lifestyle. Lack of motivation is what has allowed the pharmaceutical industry to become a multi-billion dollar industry. The idea of taking a pill and still being healthy no matter what else we eat, drink, or do, is very enticing. The idea, however, is just like the fountain of youth. If it existed, that would be great, and it would cure lots of problems. However, it's an elaborate farce. This particular farce is aimed at making money and creating power for the pharmaceutical companies.

Qualifications

Some professions may lack a governing body or qualifications to practice and, as a result, may allow practitioners who have clouded intentions, are unsafe, or are modern-day snake oil salesmen to practice. The way to prevent this is to ensure that they are qualified to practice. If not, check references for others experiences with them. If you can't find anyone well qualified, then proceed cautiously. If they don't gel with you, then find another practitioner. Even with practitioners who need qualifications (Eastern or Western-based medicines), being able to memorize for a test doesn't mean that you are honest, caring, or have the best intentions.

SECTION 3

NEW ADVANCES CONVERGING EASTERN/ WESTERN MEDICINE

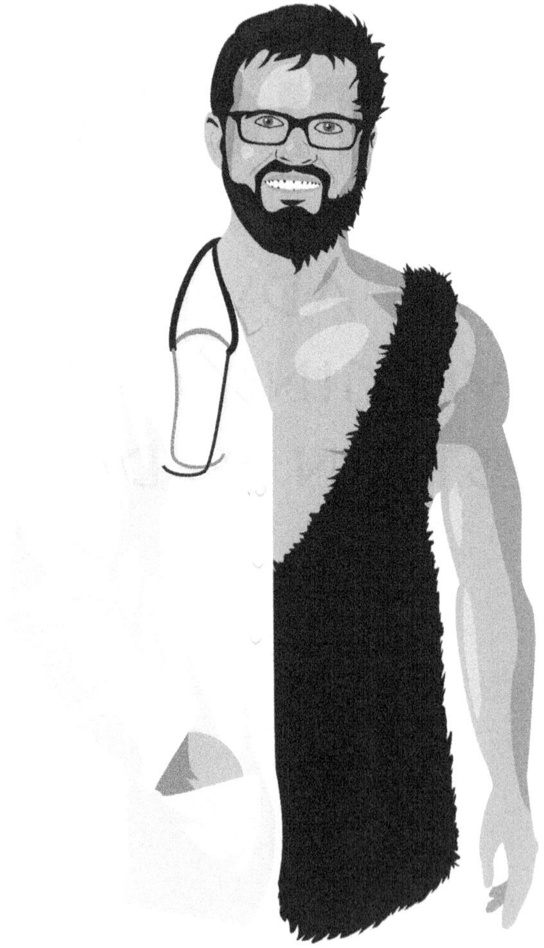

CHAPTER 7

FUNCTIONAL MEDICINE

Understands epigenetics

The field of epigenetics has emerged since we finished the human genome project. As we discovered more about human genes, we realized that, outside of a few gene mutations, the focus should be on gene expression. Gene expression is how our body decides to turn on or off certain genes based on our lifestyle and environment.

"Although there is no uniform definition of epigenetics, it has been described as heritable changes in gene function that occur without a change in the nucleotide sequence. Epigenetic modifications can be passed from one cell generation to the next (mitotic inheritance) and between generations of a species (meiotic inheritance). In plants, it is well established that epigenetic modifications can be inherited from one generation to the next. However, there is only limited information about the inheritance of epigenetic traits between generations in animals. Notably, epigenetic effects may also be affected by the environment, making them potentially important pathogenic mechanisms in complex multifactorial diseases such as type 2 diabetes. Epigenetic factors include DNA methylations, histone modifications, and microRNAs, and they can help to explain how cells with identical DNA can differentiate into different cell types with different phenotypes."[1]

http://www.ncbi.nlm.nih.gov/pmc/articles/PMC2780862/

To translate the definition above, Type 2 diabetes (DM2) may run in your family. Your genes may be more susceptible to expressing themselves in such a way that your pancreas can't handle as much sugar and carbohydrates as your neighbour. That can't be changed. But we forget the obvious solution to this issue. Stop eating sugar, grains, or processed carbs, which are all forms of glucose. The pancreas can easily process the glucose load when there is no glucose other than the appropriate amount we get from vegetables.

Think of a basement that is flooding because a water main broke. You'll probably buy a water pump to remove the water, and you might even get a bucket and carry out the water. But if you don't shut off the water main, the basement will continue flooding no matter what you do. The water is glucose in this analogy, and if you continue eating it, then you may be "unlucky" enough to have the genes for diabetes to turn on.

Later in the book, I will discuss Pottenger's Cats, which is an animal study focusing on the effects of food on chronic and degenerative diseases. The cats who ate the most processed and cooked foods had the most diseases, and the cats who ate raw, unprocessed food had virtually no chronic and degenerative diseases. If you don't believe this principle, go into a Walmart or The Warehouse and people-watch. The lowest socioeconomic classes, who have eaten the worst foods for the longest time, have the poorest health. There are obviously outliers to this observation, but, generally speaking, it is true. Once you have seen enough, go back and watch the Pottenger's Cats video. The video helps make sense of what is happening in the Western world.

Functional lab ranges vs. disease ranges

A functional lab range assesses your levels compared to the ideal, while traditional lab ranges assess compared to disease levels. I'll use the adrenal glands as my primary example. Medicine is great at assessing and treating Addison's disease and Cushing syndrome, which result from excessive or deficient cortisol levels.

Cortisol is an important hormone in your body, and is very sensitive to stress, food, and injuries, making it easy to disrupt the circadian rhythm in everyday life. Testing salivary cortisol levels through different periods of the day can determine how efficiently the adrenal gland is functioning. Most organs can be tested in different fluids or have extra tests to increase the likelihood of illuminating the issue.

Patients stating they have had their thyroid tested by their M.D./G.P., and the traditional blood tests came back normal, are a daily occurrence. Yet, they are still exhausted, cold, rundown, and just don't feel right. The tests come back normal because they don't test for optimal function. They test for complete dysfunction, and anything better than that is considered normal.

The answer to this problem is, not to get mad at those who are doing their job well, treating disease, but rather, go to the people who test for optimal function, and treat to return you to optimal function. According to Einstein, "The definition of insanity is doing the same thing over and over again, and expecting different results." If you continue to go to medical doctors to become healthy and walk away unhappy, Einstein may consider you crazy. There are many companies who test for optimal function throughout the different organ systems of the body. Your practitioner of functional medicine can help with those tests. Whether it is urine metabolites, fecal analysis, saliva, hair, or functional bloods, there are companies that exist to test these ranges.

Chapter 8

Chiropractic

Chiropractors are the ideal primary care physician for a health conscious patient. A D.C. (Doctor of Chiropractic) undergoes the same basic coursework as an M.D. (Doctor of Medicine). The main difference between the two groups of practitioners is that chiropractors focus on chiropractic adjustments, nutrition, and a holistic approach to health, while medical doctors focus on pharmaceuticals, surgeries, and intervening in a disease process. Both are necessary. However, when you present to an M.D. and they confirm that nothing is wrong, then you are often prescribed a pill. The absence of a disease process does not mean you are healthy; that is why you originally visited the doctor. Medical doctors are set up for crises and they are great at that, so let them focus on that.

While I wouldn't recommend going to a chiropractor for a prostate exam, pap smear, gunshot wound, heart attack, or venomous snake bite, I will continue to argue that chiropractors are the ideal health-oriented, primary care physician. Every day I hear several people say that they don't like taking meds, and then they rattle off a list of several that they are taking. They act as if the drugs were the only option presented.

One way to truly avoid the cabinet full of drugs is to use a primary care physician whose first objective is to fix the ailment, naturally and safely. When you use a D.C. who has the same basic educational background as your current primary care physician, you have the security of knowing that if the ailment has reached a disease process, you will be referred to the appropriate practitioner.

Most people don't realize the intensive education that is needed to become a chiropractor. I often hear jokes about the weekend certificate needed to become a chiropractor or that chiropractors aren't "real" doctors. I laugh along with these jokes as I realize no ill will is intended. But through those jokes, I am enlightened to society's continued misconceptions around the chiropractic profession. Before you read this book, did you know that chiropractors are actually primary care physicians? M.D.s do undergo an extensive residency program after graduation from school to assist in their training.

The four main aspects of a chiropractic education are the admission requirements to get into chiropractic school, the chiropractic school curriculum, board examinations, and continuing education. The four aspects of a chiropractic education are laid out more extensively in Appendix A at the back of the book.

Overview and Comparison between D.C.s, M.D.s, and P.T.s

Curriculum Requirements For the Doctor of Chiropractic Degree (DC) in comparison to the Doctor of Medicine Degree (MD) and the Doctor of Physical Therapy (DPT)

	Average Program Length	Average Classroom and Clinical Study Hours Prior to Graduation*	Advanced Certification Available
Chiropractic Curriculum	4 years	4,820	Yes
Medical Curriculum	4 years	4,670	Yes
Physical Therapy Curriculum	3 years	3,398	Yes

*Does not include hours attributed to post-graduation residency programs.

Section 4

Paleolithic Diet

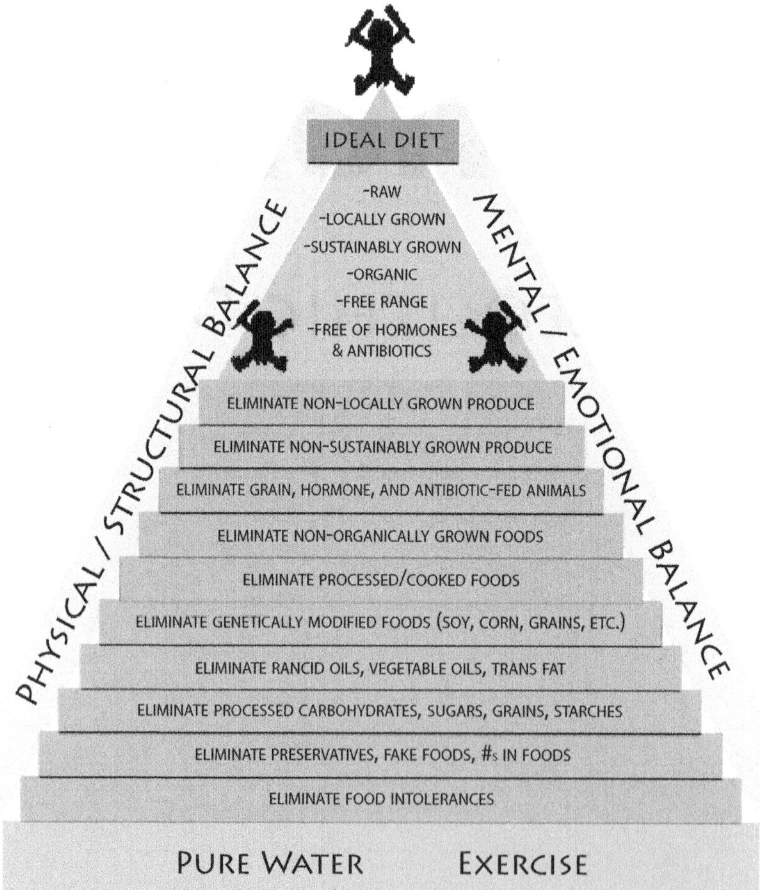
IDEAL DIET
-RAW
-LOCALLY GROWN
-SUSTAINABLY GROWN
-ORGANIC
-FREE RANGE
-FREE OF HORMONES & ANTIBIOTICS
PHYSICAL / STRUCTURAL BALANCE
MENTAL / EMOTIONAL BALANCE
ELIMINATE NON-LOCALLY GROWN PRODUCE
ELIMINATE NON-SUSTAINABLY GROWN PRODUCE
ELIMINATE GRAIN, HORMONE, AND ANTIBIOTIC-FED ANIMALS
ELIMINATE NON-ORGANICALLY GROWN FOODS
ELIMINATE PROCESSED/COOKED FOODS
ELIMINATE GENETICALLY MODIFIED FOODS (SOY, CORN, GRAINS, ETC.)
ELIMINATE RANCID OILS, VEGETABLE OILS, TRANS FAT
ELIMINATE PROCESSED CARBOHYDRATES, SUGARS, GRAINS, STARCHES
ELIMINATE PRESERVATIVES, FAKE FOODS, #s IN FOODS
ELIMINATE FOOD INTOLERANCES
PURE WATER
EXERCISE
CHEMICAL / NUTRITIONAL BALANCE

Chapter 9

What is the Paleo Diet?

The Paleolithic diet is simple: Eat like we did 10,000 to 5,000,000 years ago because the last 10,000 years isn't what we are meant to be eating. Before we started farming, we had the exact same food supply throughout human evolutionary history. It's a concept that's simple to grasp, tricky at times to implement, and undeniably the most logical diet.

Let's look into why the paleo diet argues that our genetics have not yet adapted to these new foods. Science believes that the evolutionary history of mankind started 5 million years ago. Let's assume that a new generation comes along every 20 years (reproduce at age 20). Based off these assumptions, 249,500 generations (4,990,000 years) of cavemen before you and I had the exact same food supply and evolved from Homo habilis to Homo sapiens.

Over the last 500 generations (10,000 years), we have started to introduce these man-made foods and find it absurd that they could still be causing problems. Over the past 80 years, we have started adding pesticides and herbicides to our fields to kill pests and weeds that hurt these plants. The plants no longer have to defend themselves from pests or compete for nutrients with the weeds, which makes them much weaker than their spray-free counterparts.

We are now in our fourth generation of evolution adversely affected by sprays. Recombinant DNA technology was created in the 1970s and first used in the 1980s. This is at the center of the genetically modified organism (GMO) debate that is so controversial. What recombinant DNA technology allows is for humans to splice genes and create foods that wouldn't exist in nature. Add this into the human evolutionary process for the last two generations.

In summary:

249,500 generations; same food supply

500 generations; farming and processing dramatically alters food supply

4 generations; chemicals and sprays that kill plant life and insects applied in vast quantities to our food supply

2 generations; using viral DNA to create GMO crops that wouldn't otherwise exist

CHAPTER 10

PROS OF PALEO

The paleo diet gets us back to the basic foods that have been around as long as our evolution as a species.

Vegetables

Vegetables would have been a steady source of nutrition to our Paleolithic ancestors. There would've been an abundance of leafy greens available during the spring and summer months, gourds and sweet potatoes were available from fall into midwinter, along with a variety of other vegetables sprouting throughout the year. We'd have been surrounded with delicious, fresh, locally grown, sustainably grown, 100% organic, spray-free, seasonal vegetables for most of the year. We wouldn't have fried, battered, or boiled them to remove the nutrition from them.

Soy is eliminated

Soy needs to be eliminated from your diet at all costs because, along with corn and wheat, it's one of the most genetically modified and heavily processed foods. Whether as TVP, soy lecithin, soy milk, or soy flour, we have created a problematic food as devastating to our health as gluten, and yet we portray it as a health food. Soy is one of the three foods that I see in my practice most commonly associated with thyroid and reproductive issues. The isoflavones in soy are what we think is responsible for the goitrogenic effect on the thyroid, along with the estrogenic effects on the female reproductive system.

Let's look at the soy plant today compared to 100 years ago. Soy is a very big industry, and creating higher yields each year is the name of the game. This happens through genetically modifying the plants to create more beans per plant, with fewer nutrients in the soil than we had 100 years ago. As we continue to genetically modify these foods, we change the effects these foods have on us.

The most common response I get when I tell people to avoid soy is, "No big deal, I don't eat it anyway." To which I respond, "That's what everyone says. Read all of your labels and if it says soy lecithin, lecithin, vegetable oil, brominated vegetable oil, soy milk, soy flour, tofu, or emulsifier # anything—you need to avoid it." On the second visit, they always come back a little angry and say, "I can't eat anything." We then share a laugh, and I tell them which of their favorite foods they can find in a soy-free version. The biggest difficulty is usually chocolate, but not to worry, there are soy-free chocolates available.

Fruits

Fruit was another regular part of a Paleolithic diet, from apples to strawberries and everything in between. Each fruit had a shorter window of availability, as each fruit ripens during a particular time frame. But there would have been an abundance of each fruit for a short period of time. We would have eaten large amounts of these fruits during this short time and only during this time. But these fruits would have been fresh, locally grown, sustainably grown, seasonal, and 100% organic and spray-free.

Meat

Meat of many varieties would have been eaten in Paleolithic times; however, it would have been consumed much differently today. When your only weapon is a sharpened rock, stick, or your bare hands, hunting for red meat like deer, elk, buffalo, bear, cow, or sheep would have been more dangerous than hunting for chicken, fish, or turkey. During the months when chicken, fish, and turkey were available, we would have eaten them instead of putting ourselves in danger hunting the more dangerous animals. During the late winter months, as fish were already unavailable due to the freezing of lakes, and the fowl population decreased as the weak died, we would have been forced to hunt more dangerous animals.

After a successful hunt, we would eat the most nutritious parts of the animal, and we would have eaten lots of it. The most nutritious parts are the organs, namely the kidneys, adrenals, liver, heart, etc. We would have left most of the rest of the muscle tissue for the scavengers because muscle is void of nutrition in comparison to the incredibly nutrient-rich organs.

The problem with eating organs of modern day animals is the toxic strain of modern-day society. The liver processes toxins in our body, and gets them ready for excretion; the kidney excretes the toxins, along with the intestines. The adrenal glands deal with stress, and living in crowded feedlots creates an unnatural stress response in animals, The heart is damaged by excess sugar, and yet we feed these animals corn and grains that break down into glucose—a.k.a. sugar!

The safest portion of meat in today's world is the, comparatively speaking, nutritionally deficient muscle that would have been left for scavengers because we had no real way to thaw the frozen meat, (frozen during winter) or to prevent spoiling during warmer weather. This would have curbed our hunger for a period, until the hunger overcame the danger we perceived, and we decided to hunt instead of starve.

Let's say that you are determined to get good organ meat; what do you have to do? You need to find meat, raised free-range, with no hormones or antibiotics. This helps create organs more suitable to be consumed. The toxins in our environment are still getting into the animals, so if you own your animals, try to have wild herbs growing like milk thistle, horsetail, burdock root, and broccoli sprouts that help support phase 1 and 2 detoxification in the animal's liver. Doing this would allow for most of the animals organs to be much safer to consume. Alternatively, soaking the organs in lemon juice will help bind and eliminate many toxins that managed to get into the organ.

How often should you eat red meat? Some say it should be avoided altogether. Some say it should be avoided except for once a week, or even once a month. I say it should be eaten more in the winter, when our ancestors would have eaten it (although they would have eaten meat during droughts and famines as well). To test how often you need red meat, try not eating red meat for a few weeks to a month. See how long it takes you to start thinking about grabbing a pocket knife, jumping the fence, and killing the scary looking bull because your need for meat is so intense that your animal instinct is overriding the danger associated with attacking a much larger, stronger, faster animal.

For me, that period in winter is around three to four weeks. I may eat it more frequently than that because I get irritable after a week or two, and I need to be tolerant for work. This is mostly from the instinctive behaviours, developed through the previous 249,500 generations (4,990,000 years) of cavemen before me who lived this way, and the last 500 generations (10,000 years) have not bred that out of my genes (instincts) yet. The answer to how often you should eat red meat is different for everyone, but this technique is one way you can assess how often is right for you.

CHAPTER 11

CONS OF PALEO DIET

Through our all-knowing intelligence, humans have completely changed our food supply over the past 10,000 years from hunter-gatherer to farmer. Over the past 100 years, it has become much worse as technology has advanced. Instead of allowing nature to naturally select which form of soy, corn, grain, and vegetables will thrive, we create forms of food in a lab using viral DNA technologies (recombinant DNA technology), inject them with poisons so bugs don't eat the genetic abominations, harvest them, and transport them to a factory where they then process these foods having no actual nutritional value that isn't artificially added, and then hundreds of millions of dollars are spent on marketing to get you to believe, buy, and consume their verbal and culinary garbage.

Primal diet

The primal diet is a form of the paleo diet that allows dairy, one of the three most problematic foods (dairy, gluten, soy) to be consumed by humans. Just like soy and gluten, dairy goes through a large amount of processing that changes it from the raw form that may possibly carry any health benefits. However, even in its raw form, humans aren't meant to drink cow's milk—calves are.

This diet will be almost as much work as the paleo diet, and you may get none of the results because dairy causes so many of its own problems for a large proportion of people. An argument of the pros and cons of dairy would fill a book, so I will focus on the logic behind who would consume dairy.

Historically, only one animal is meant to consume an animal's milk and that is the offspring who caused the lactation to occur. It would be much more logical and healthy to milk humans. A human's milk is meant to turn a child into a full-grown human, while a cow's milk turns a calf into a cow. If humans drink cow's milk, do we become cattle? Not exactly, but we do put on a lot of extra weight and have several other side effects. This is why whey protein is used in protein powders. The next time you feel you are meant to consume dairy, chase that mother cow through the field, hang upside down, and latch on to the udder and enjoy!

It is quite simple to change a primal diet into a paleo diet by substituting coconut oil for butter, coconut ice cream for ice cream, coconut yogurt for yogurt, and coconut-almond-hemp or hazelnut milks for dairy milk. The dairy supporter will then sarcastically say, "Was coconut milk around 10,000 years ago?" The answer is no, but coconuts were, and we would have been able to consume them.

Genetic alterations to foods

Humans have dramatically changed the natural state of many foods, by genetically modifying their genes with viruses to optimize yields, minimize insect destruction of crops, and eliminate those annoying seeds that impede our ability to inhale the food.

This makes it impossible for us to eat exactly like our Paleolithic ancestors. But eating a raw banana that has been modified to remove all of the seeds is better than eating rice cakes, a piece of bread, luncheon meat, or cheese. The only reason I touch on this thought is to address the argument by some of the anti-paleo types.

There are people out there in the scientific community who are trying to make a difference and protect our food supply and our health. One specific organization called the Bio-Protection Research Center looks into ways to protect crops without harmful pesticides, herbicides, or fungicides. They also look at the efficacy of GMO crops. Here are a few links to papers to help understand more about the health and environmental impact of these practices.

http://bioprotection.org.nz/research/innovative-bioprotection

http://bit.ly/22Y3dPY

Section 5

Paleolithic Doctor

The Paleolithic doctor will focus on lifestyle modifications first. This involves promoting exercise, eating naturally, fresh air, plenty of sunshine, and clean water. Obviously, a Paleolithic doctor will promote the Paleolithic diet in some form as a main lifestyle recommendation, but also exercising outdoors to help the other main requirements of the diet.

This is the very basic element that all Paleolithic doctors should know. They should have a working understanding of disease processes and medical emergencies, so no matter what office a patient goes to, whether it be an M.D. (medical doctor), D.O. (osteopath), D.C. (chiropractor), D.D.S. (dentist), or any other doctor, they will be assured that their case will be handled correctly and referred out if necessary.

I will use myself as an example of this principle. As a chiropractor and certified nutrition specialist, my primary treatment is still finding the lifestyle source of the problem, if one exists, and first altering that behavior, thought, emotion, toxin, or food. Along with that lifestyle alteration, I utilize chiropractic adjustments to correct bony malpositions and, if needed, nutritional supplements to help promote the natural healing process.

The Paleolithic doctor should be willing to work with all types of other practitioners, regardless of the credentials, based on the quality of the practitioner and not on the prejudices of a degree. Two of the best ways for patients and practitioners alike to find a doctor who practices this way are the following websites:

www.primaldocs.com

www.paleophysiciansnetwork.com

CHAPTER 12

MODIFIED PALEO DIET

The Paleolithic doctor is what the doctor of the future should be. They need to practice a form of the Paleolithic diet and promote a healthy lifestyle. They need a working understanding of both Eastern and Western medicine, meaning that they need to understand the concept of an energetic aspect to the body in whichever form you want to call it.

They should know how to apply the appropriate manual or energetic therapies as needed. It is very important that they understand the disease processes of different conditions and are able to identify red flags that need to be referred out. They should stress the importance of exercise in your daily routine, and they need at least a basic understanding of nutrition to keep you healthy in a world with an ever worsening food supply.

Most importantly, they need to promote that everything about your food matters, including where it is grown, how it is grown (sustainably vs. new age farming, high NPK, etc.), organic vs. inorganic, raw vs. cooked, if cooked then how, and what food pyramid you use.

Here is my version of a paleo diet that also leaves common food intolerances out of the paleo/primal diet. I have included a few non-paleo cheats that are handy during the transitional period between a normal Western diet and the Paleolithic diet that will only affect hormonal balance (glucose balancing forces hormonal changes in body) in most people.

Dairy (milk, cheese, yogurt, casein)

Gluten (bread, baked goods, packaged products, barley, bulgur, dinkle, durum, couscous (wheat variety), einkorn, faro, graham flour, khorasan, matza (matzah, matzo), mir, rye, semolina, spelt, triticale)

Coffee (if gluten-free diet, no coffee because it can react like gluten in some people) (10% of population)

Oats (has a molecule similar to gluten that reacts the same in a percentage of people)

Soy (lecithin (added in chocolate), tofu, soy milk, soy sauce, tamari, vegetable oil, soybean oil, brominated vegetable oil)

Corn (chips, on the cob, canned, bread, high fructose corn syrup, corn syrup, corn oil, maltodextrin)

All GMO food (our bodies don't recognize most of these "frankenfoods")

Eating food raw is how we were meant to eat it, so when possible, consume raw vegetables, mixed nuts, fruits, and seeds. Cook meats to safe temperatures.

The second most important part of diet, see Pottenger's Cats argument in Chapter 13.

Organic, locally grown produce is best; organic, regionally grown is second best; organic is third best; non-organic is fourth best (all non-GMO).

Cut all pop/soda/fizzy drinks out of your diet. Diet/zero-cal/no-sugar is even worse than regular pop because fake sugars like aspartame are suspected neurotoxins, and we don't know the extent of the harm they cause.

Consume ½ your body weight (in lbs) in ounces of clean ((spring or artesian water bottled in an area not close to a major city) water daily (more with heavy workout or sweating). 108 oz is sufficient for a 216-lb individual (1-oz of water per kg) 1 liter is equal to 34 ounces.

Lemon wedge, lime wedge, cucumber slice, mint leaves are good additions to water and provide variety.

Use high-quality, pink, Himalayan salt (85 trace minerals) when needed instead of table salt (iodized sodium chloride).

Sample Diet

Wake up

Drink a 24-oz glass of clean water first thing (lemon wedge optional)

Take shower, get ready for work, etc.

Eat breakfast

(Eating a good source of protein is vital for energy production during your entire day.)

2 to 3 eggs (free-range and organic is best) (poached is best)

2 to 3 strips of bacon (or equivalent amount of other meats) (grass-fed, organic is best)(nitrate/nitrite free)

> Broil (grill) in oven.
>
> The nitrite/nitrate free part is the most important. Sodium and potassium nitrate and nitrite are the preservatives largely responsible for increased rates of colon cancer in meat eaters. It's not the meat itself that is the problem.

Look for them as preservatives #249-252 on the label.

(Bacon is a motivator to get you switched to the paleo diet. Once you are fully into the diet, replace with chicken, steak, fish, etc.)

Piece of fruit

Apple
Pear
Banana

Non-processed carbohydrate

Cut up a whole kumara/ sweet potato (cook it with the eggs and bacon)

Beverage

Clean water (12 oz)Herbal tea (no caffeine)

Almond milk, coconut milk, flax milk, hemp milk, rice milk (**all unsweetened**)

Green tea (least amount of caffeine of 3 choices here)

Black tea (middle amount of caffeine of 3 choices here)

Juice

Coffee (most amount of caffeine of 3 choices here) *No coffee if you're on a gluten-free diet because it can react like gluten in some people.

Or a shake in the morning (time-saver and healthy)

Almond milk, coconut milk, flax milk, hemp milk, rice milk

Condensed fruits and vegetables powder (or blended veggies)

Protein, fiber, essential fatty acids
*No whey protein, or casein (dairy-based adds weight on)
*No soy protein

2 to 3 tbsp of chia seeds (ground)
7.5 g of carbohydrates, 5 g of fat, and 2.5 g of protein, lots of heart-healthy omega-3 fatty acids, 2 g of fiber

2 to 3 tbsp of hemp hearts
5 g of total fat, 1 g of saturated fat, 4 g of polyunsaturated fat, 1 mg of sodium, 1 g of carbohydrates, 1 g of dietary fiber, 4 g of protein and 8% of the daily recommended value of calcium, also contain vitamin A, vitamin C, vitamin D, vitamin E, and B vitamins.

Essential fatty acids

Grind 2 to 3 tbsp of flax seeds (golden or brown, both work)

Fiber

Psyllium husk
Slippery elm

Slow and prolonged absorption of healthy carbs (in small amounts) at breakfast improves the glycemic response after lunch (prevents mid-afternoon tiredness)

We achieve this by eating small amounts of carbs (in the form of vegetables) with fat and protein.

Why should I avoid eating cereal, oatmeal, biscuits, donuts, etc. for breakfast and have protein instead? I heard having meat and eggs were bad for my cholesterol. This is a very common question I hear from patients. The answer is very complex, but I will give the abbreviated version here.

A good resource to help educate you more on this topic is *The Great Cholesterol Myth* by Johnny Bowden.

When you eat a processed carbohydrate for breakfast, you highly elevate your blood sugar (carbs get broken down to glucose, which is a form of sugar), and you get a sudden energy burst that makes you feel good. We call that the "high" from sugar. Your body responds to this high level of sugar in the blood stream by releasing insulin, which takes the damaging glucose molecule and deposits it into fat cells, increasing fat production. In response to the lack of energy available from the insulin surge, your adrenal gland will release cortisol, which makes glucose available for the body. This process goes back and forth and is what is responsible for the sugar cravings we experience. It is also responsible for the fatigue you may feel around 2:00 p.m. to 3:00 p.m.

Sugar (glucose) is damaging to the arteries and veins, which is why our body does its best to regulate the levels in a narrow range. But we place too great a demand on the body with high-carbohydrate/sugar consumption and it can't keep up. The glucose then damages the arterial lining, which is where cholesterol comes into play. Cholesterol is your body's way of fixing the damage created by the glucose in our arteries.

Picture your arteries as a house. The glucose is like a fire in the house. If it's contained within the fireplace, then it is in control and good. If it gets out of control and starts a house fire, the cholesterol puts out the fire (the firefighter).

To lower your cholesterol, you should decrease the need for it by getting rid of the glucose. Otherwise, artificially lowering your cholesterol is like shooting the firefighters who are putting out the house fire.

Fueling Your Body (Fireplace Analogy)

Eating a breakfast high in protein and low in processed carbs will create long-lasting energy with no sugar regulation issues. Imagine a fireplace that heats your house. In this analogy, your metabolism is the fire. Protein and fats are the logs of your metabolism, while carbohydrates are like paper. If you only throw a bunch of paper in the fireplace and walk away to do other things, the fire will go out because the paper burns so fast. We all know logs burn for a long time an produce a steady, even heat. You are free to focus on other activities because the fire continues to burn for a long time.

Morning snack

(No processed carbs!)

Choices

Mixed nuts (raw, unsalted)
Vegetables
Berries
Beef jerky (low-processed, no gluten, dairy, or soy)

Beverage

Clean water (12 oz)
Tea
Kombucha

Lunch

Vegetables

Kale
Broccoli
Green beans
Spinach
Asparagus
Green peas
Bell peppers (assorted colors)
Tomatoes (technically a fruit but allowed)
Cucumbers
Kumara (sweet potato)
Cauliflower

Beans (middle portion) (not paleo)

Based off of blood type recommendations. Vegans often rely on legumes to get protein. (Not paleo diet-approved, but some people can't do without, and I'm reasonable while starting the diet.)

Blood type O
aduke, adzuki, pinto, black-eyed

Blood type A
aduke, adzuki, black, green, pinto, red and green lentils, black-eyed peas

Blood type B
kidney, lima, navy

Blood type AB
navy, pinto, red and green lentils

Lean meat (middle portion)

Grass-fed chicken
Grass-fed beef

Unprocessed carbs
(smallest portion) (not paleo approved, but mostly non-allergenic)

Brown rice
Wild rice
Quinoa

Beverage

Clean water (12 oz)
Herbal tea
Kombucha

Afternoon snack

Mixed nuts (raw, unsalted)

Berries

Vegetables

Beverage

Clean water (12 oz)
Herbal or root tea
Kombucha

Dinner

Vegetables

Kale
Broccoli
Green beans
Spinach
Asparagus
Green peas
Bell peppers
Tomatoes
Cucumbers
Squash
Sweet potato

Lean meat (small amount)

Unprocessed carbohydrates
(smallest amounts) (not paleo approved)

Brown rice
Wild rice
Potato

Beverage

Clean water (24 oz)
Kombucha

***If having alcohol:**

Hard alcohol (up to 2 servings for adult male, 1 serving for female) (a serving is 1.5 ounces)

Red wine (2 servings for adult male, 1 serving for female)

Hard cider (2 servings for adult male, 1 serving for female)

Late-night snack

Vegetables

Mixed nuts (raw, unsalted) (good due to trace minerals that help with sleep)

Beverage

Clean water (12 oz)
Herbal or root tea

Food	Approve	Not the worst choice	Disapprove
Vegetables	all fresh vegetables	potatoes/ carrots	
Fruits	most fresh fruits	tomatoes, dried fruits	
Animal products	chicken, fish, beef, lamb, pork		if they contain preservatives
Nuts	raw nuts	roasted nuts	roasted and covered with sugary substance, peanuts (see legumes)
Oils (in moderation)	animal fats, coconut oil, olive oil		vegetable oils (corn, soy, etc.)
Legumes	-	correct blood type approved	peanuts
Grains	-	-	all
Dairy	-	-	all
Other	honey, maple syrup		preservatives, numbered food, artificial sweeteners, sugar

CHAPTER 13

POTTENGER'S CATS

A perfect example of an Eastern vs. Western approach to health, and how everything about food matters, is Pottenger's Cats. Pottenger's Cats was an experiment on cats carried out during part of the first half of the 19th century. The study focused on the effect of diet on chronic and degenerative disease, comparing the effects of raw vs. cooked meat and viscera, as well as processed vs. unprocessed milk. The results of this study were staggering and varied from perfect health, in the raw unprocessed fed diet four generations after the start of the experiment, to the infertility and massive amount of degenerative disease in the cooked and processed food group.
(https://www.youtube.com/watch?v=XPCOGSnjP5w)

One argument against the study's results is that the experiment isn't applicable because cats don't represent humans well. Another argument is that the taurine was cooked out of the food and that was responsible for all of the various diseases.

In defense of the study, humans are animals just like cats are. We may be affected in a different manner than cats, but we are still affected. Because our lifespans are much longer than cats, it takes longer for changes to appear. And these changes are starting to appear. The simple lesson that is often missed is that animals are affected by their food. Everything matters, from what we eat to how it's prepared. The old saying, "You are what you eat," made sense to many generations before ours, but somehow we have lost that understanding.

The taurine argument is a minimalistic look at the argument made by Pottenger. We know from basic chemistry that the way to create a chemical reaction is to add heat, pressure, or a chemical reagent. Heating food creates chemical reactions that change the nutrition in the food.

As a society, we don't fully understand all of the functions of even one of the more than 25,000 phytonutrients we know exist. Who thinks we know all the effects of any of the reactive products created from cooking the food and altering the phytonutrient content?

If this isn't enough to convince you, or if it scares you too much, never fear. Look to the American population to see what this food alteration can do (which is a much scarier version of Pottenger's Cats). Some are more susceptible than others, thanks to epigenetics and biochemical individuality, but we are all vulnerable to some extent. Pottenger's Cats also demonstrated that returning to a raw diet could reverse some of the effects.

CHAPTER 14

WHY YOUR DOCTOR NEEDS TO BE TRAINED IN WESTERN MEDICINE

Western medicine has done a great job of identifying the disease process and diagnosing you appropriately. The treatment of diseases like ALS, Parkinson's, and Huntington's Disease, are examples of knowing what the disease is, and as a result, knowing what to expect from it.

This approach will also allow for drugs to alleviate some of these symptoms.

The problem with this approach is that we don't know what causes the disease. We are heading down a path where we believe diet and lifestyle don't matter because it is all due to your genetics.

A perfect example of this are lifestyle diseases like Type 2 diabetes, metabolic syndrome, and high cholesterol that are controlled by prescribing an ever-increasing amount of drugs. There is minimal patient education on correct diets to prevent these conditions, and an ever-increasing number of drugs for each ailment. A sign warning us of the curve ahead is much more useful than an ambulance at the bottom of the cliff. It's even better than a multi-billion-dollar hospital with the best emergency room, surgeons, and drugs.

Western medicine is also great in medical emergencies. This includes, but is not limited to, broken bones, gunshot wounds, stab wounds, anaphylactic shock, internal bleeding, and heart attacks. Emergency medicine is perfect on the course it is heading in.

CHAPTER 15

WHY YOUR DOCTOR NEEDS TO BE TRAINED IN EASTERN MEDICINE

Eastern medicine has done a great job of maintaining health. Over 6,000 years of practice have proven that acupuncture, herbal medicine, and chiropractic adjustments, among other treatments, are beneficial for maintaining health.

An important part of life is not forgetting what has worked well in the past. With the failing health of the average American and all citizens of the Western world, the American and global population is starting to realize that pharmaceutical companies, insurance companies, and the medical establishment don't have all the answers. We need to stop believing the marketing of multi-billion-dollar companies like Monsanto, GlaxoSmithKline, Coca-Cola, Kellogg's, the Dairy Coalition, and government-funded corporate partners who have mastered the art of marketing to sell their products. The problem for Eastern medicine is that there isn't a hundred-billion-dollar a year industry supporting it, and as a result, it remains vilified and out of the public eye.

My Final Message

I want to leave you with a personal message from a man who has first-hand experience with what we refer to as "bad luck." In my case, bad luck was also called a pineal germinoma.

Bad Luck

I want you to picture the most grand casinos you have ever seen with marble floors, bright lights, and thousands of people. How do casinos afford to be so flashy? Bad luck? No. That is laughable, and we usually ridicule the person who says they had bad luck at the casino. Statistics are the reason the casino is so fancy. The odds are stacked in favor of the house, and the casino wins every day.

I want you to now picture a big fancy hospital with marble floors, bright lights, cutting edge technologies, and thousands of people each day going through the revolving doors. Why are so many people getting diabetes, cancer, degenerative diseases, and gene polymorphisms and mutations? Bad luck?

That is the answer we still accept, but it's no less laughable than the scenario in the casino described above. The reasoning has not changed; statistics are still to blame. If you eat enough processed garbage food, you are more likely to have "bad luck." If you don't exercise regularly, you are more likely to have "bad luck." If you surround yourself with electronic devices during all waking hours, you are more likely to have "bad luck." If you do all of these things, then you're much more likely to have "bad luck."

I was fortunate to have Western medicine to help me. However, if I'm presented with the challenge of having cancer again, I am convinced I would decline and undergo different treatments outside of chemotherapy, radiation, brain surgery, and countless drugs. While I am grateful to be alive, vomiting 30+ times a day from the effects of chemotherapy, taking 20 different types of strong medications, breaking out in hives from drug reactions, having infected surgery scars, plus many more challenges, are things I don't wish to ever face again. Only time and "bad luck" will prove if that's a decision I will have to make.

Preventing cancer, metabolic syndrome, diabetes, and heart disease, are some of the biggest challenges facing our generation. As cancer rates continue to rise, we are forced to ask what the cause is. While no one cause is responsible, our modern lifestyle, from food all the way to modern technology, is a definite contributor. Becoming more like our caveman ancestors is a step to preventing our own health challenges. The next time you see a multi-billion dollar pharmaceutical company doing a fundraiser for cancer research, I challenge you to get inspired to be as caveman as you can be in our modern world.

To find more content from Dr. Carl Bamlet, you can find him on Facebook at Dr. Carl Bamlet: The Modern Caveman, listen to live streaming of his radio show on 96.9 plainsfm, or watch his television program on CTV or at yumpaleo.com.

Dr. Bamlet is available for consults in both the United States and New Zealand at the following locations:

United States

15th December – 15th January

Pirkl Chiropractic
2711 Commerce Dr. NW # 300
Rochester, MN 55901

New Zealand

16th January – 14th December

The Alpha Omega Clinic
66 Innes Rd, St Albans
Christchurch 8052

Paleo Recipes

PALEO APPLE PIE

CRUST INGREDIENTS

3 cups almond flour

½ cup coconut oil, melted

2 tsp pink, Himalayan salt

½ tsp Ceylon cinnamon

CRUST PREPARATION

In a large bowl, combine almond flour, coconut oil and salt

Mix until it takes on a doughy texture.

Cut the dough into two even chunks.

Evenly distribute one portion of dough into 9-inch pie dish.

The remaining dough is to be used as the top crust for the pie, so roll it out and set aside for later use.

FILLING INGREDIENTS

7 apples, peeled and thinly sliced

2 tbsp almond flour

½ tsp Ceylon cinnamon

¼ tsp nutmeg

2 tsp lemon juice

FILLING PREPARATION

Preheat oven to 350 F (175 C). In a large bowl, toss apples in lemon juice

In a separate smaller bowl, combine almond flour, cinnamon, and nutmeg

Pour the almond flour mixture over the apples and coat apples evenly

Take the dough prepared earlier and place it on top of the pie.

Press the edges together with the dough used to make the pie shell.

Cut small holes in the top of the crust to allow heat to escape.

Put the apple filling into the pie shell and cook for approximately 70 minutes.

PALEO BANANA BREAD

This is a delicious treat the whole family will love, and you don't need to feel guilty about it. There's no sugar or artificial sweetener, flour or grains, and is free of most allergens.

INGREDIENTS

1 cup almond flour

½ cup coconut flour

¼ cup flax seed meal (ground flax seed)

1 tsp pink, Himalayan salt

4 eggs

2 tbsp coconut oil, melted

1 tbsp maple syrup

1 tsp vanilla extract

2 large ripe banana, mashed

1/2 tsp of cinnamon

If desired, add dark chocolate/carob chips (dairy, soy, and sugar-free) in moderation. If you can't find dairy, soy, and sugar-free, don't use.

PREPARATION

Preheat oven to 350 F (175 C)

Grease 2 small loaf pans (5¾ x 3½)

Combine dry ingredients in a medium bowl

Combine wet ingredients in a small bowl and whisk together

Pour wet into dry ingredients and mix until fully incorporated

Divide evenly (dough will be thick) into loaf pans and smooth the tops

Bake for about 35 to 50 min, checking frequently

Remove loaves from oven, let cool in pans for 5 minutes, and then transfer to a wire rack or counter to continue cooling

RAW PALEO BROWNIE

Base Ingredients

4 tbsp flax seeds

4 tbsp cacao nibs

3 tbsp date paste

Juice of ½ orange

2 tbsp honey

Extra Ingredients

¼ tsp ground vanilla beans

1 tsp cinnamon

2 tbsp dried fruit (blueberries, cherries, cranberries)

Base Preparation

Grind flax seeds and cacao nibs into fine granules

Pour into mixing bowl, as well as other desired extras, and add date paste and juice of orange

Mix thoroughly

Oil or wax paper small baking dish

Evenly layer mixture into small baking dish

Spread a thin layer of honey onto the base layer

Place in oven at 375 F (200 C) for approximately 7 minutes

Topping Ingredients

1 bar homemade/unsweetened chocolate or 1 bar 85% dark chocolate (not paleo)

Topping Preparation

Place chocolate bar onto base and place in oven until chocolate melts, remove from oven

Place in refrigerator and allow chocolate to firm

PALEO POTATO SALAD

INGREDIENTS

1 medium raw orange kumara (sweet potato)

1 large raw avocado

3 large hardboiled eggs

1 to 2 tbsp dressing as desired (cold-pressed extra virgin olive oil or balsamic vinaigrette) (look for sulphite-free varieties)

1 to 5 tsp organic yellow mustard (no additives or numbers) to taste

mayonnaise, optional (must be paleo, no dairy, soy, E#'s, etc.)

salt and pepper

PREPARATION

Wash kumara and peel outer layer if non-organic, scrub off dirt while washing if organic

Chop kumara into cubes

Boil kumara in water until soft but not falling apart

Boil 3 eggs for approximately 10 minutes until yolk is hard.

The keys to having eggs that peel easy are as follows:

1. High-quality eggs
2. Place into cool water, and then boil
3. Add salt, vinegar, and baking soda to the boiling water

(Some people also find that steaming the eggs for 10 minutes instead of boiling can help with peeling.)

While the eggs and kumara boil, cut the avocado into cubes

When eggs finish boiling, run under cold water to cool and then peel

Cut the eggs into cubes (roughly 8 cubes per egg)

Add mustard and dressing

Mix everything in a large bowl

Salt and pepper to taste

RAW PALEO SLAW

INGREDIENTS

2 medium raw carrots

1 large raw beetroot

1 large raw apple

2 tbsp black currants or raisins

1 to 3 tbsp dressing (cold-pressed extra virgin olive oil or balsamic vinaigrette as desired, sulphite-free) and dash of pomegranate juice

raw or cold smoked salmonsalt and pepper

sesame seeds, sunflower seeds, or pumpkin seeds if desired

a cup of wilted spinach is a great addition to this dish

PREPARATION

Remove apple core

Wash carrot, apple, and beetroot (vinegar-based spray to remove waxes if desired)

Peel outer layer of vegetables if non-organic, scrub off dirt while washing if organic

Chop apple, carrot, and beetroot into matchstick-sizes pieces (cheese grater may be faster)

Add black currants and seed choice(s) and stir

Add dressing and stir

Salt and pepper to taste

Chop salmon into bite-sized pieces and add to dish

ROAST CHICKEN AND VEGETABLES

Ingredients

2 medium broccoli heads

1 large beetroot

1 large kumara (sweet potato)

1 to 3 tbsp dressing as desired (coconut or sunflower oil or balsamic vinaigrette)

4 free range, hormone-free chicken thighs

2 lemons

1 orange

salt and pepper

6 tbsp sesame seeds

2 tsp ground kelp

Vegetables Preparation

Wash vegetables and peel outer layer if non-organic, scrub off dirt while washing if organic

Cut vegetables into ½ -inch cubes (approximately)

Add dressing and stir

Place vegetables into baking dish

Salt and pepper as desired

Chicken Preparation

Cut and juice orange and lemons

Add juice to chicken and let sit for 30 minutes

Mix sesame seeds, kelp, pepper, and salt in a large bowl

Place chicken thighs into mixture one at a time making sure to coat both sides

Place chicken thighs on top of vegetables

COOKING

Place in oven at 375 F (200 C) for approximately 40 minutes or until chicken is crispy on the outside and juicy on the inside

Remove chicken and let it rest

Return vegetables to oven until crispy, approximately 5 to 10 minutes

CUSTARD APPLE AND BANANA PUDDING

Ingredients

2 bananas

1 large custard apple (ripe)

2 tsp Ceylon cinnamon

3 tbsp cocoa nibs

¼ cup blueberries

¼ cup raspberries

Preparation

Cut custard apple in half and remove seeds

Scrape custard apple into bowl

Peel and cut bananas

Mash bananas and add to custard apple

Add cocoa nibs to mix

Add cinnamon to mix

Mix by hand or with food processor

Add berries to bottom of two small glass bowls

Pour mix on top

ROAST BREAKFAST AND POACHED EGGS

Ingredients

2 medium broccoli heads

1 large beetroot

1 large kumara (sweet potato)

1 to 3 tbsp dressing as desired (coconut or sunflower oil or balsamic vinaigrette)

4 free-range, hormone-free chicken thighs

salt and pepper to taste

6 eggs

1 tsp apple cider vinegar

Vegetables Preparation

Wash vegetables and peel outer layer if non-organic, scrub off dirt while washing if organic

Cut vegetables into ½ -inch cubes (approximately)

Add dressing and stir

Place vegetables into baking dish

Salt and pepper to taste

Chicken Preparation

Place chicken thighs on top of vegetables

Eggs Preparation

Boil water in small sauce pan with a dash of salt and apple cider vinegar. Poach eggs 3 at a time.

Cooking

Place in oven at 375 F (200 C) for approximately 40 minutes or until chicken is crispy on the outside and juicy on the inside

Remove chicken and let it rest

Start poaching eggs and return vegetables to oven until crispy, approximately 5 to10 min

PALEO FISH WITH SALT AND VINEGAR CHIPS

Ingredients

2 large kumara (sweet potatoes)

1 to 3 tbsp dressing as desired (coconut or sunflower oil or balsamic vinaigrette)

2 fish fillets of desired fish

salt and pepper to taste

apple cider vinegar

4 tbsp of sesame seeds

4 tbsp of flaxseeds

Chips Preparation

Wash kumara and peel outer layer if non-organic, scrub off dirt while washing if organic

Cut kumara into desired size

Drizzle with apple cider vinegar and oil

Place vegetables onto baking sheet

Salt and pepper as desired

Fish Preparation

Grind sesame and flax seeds and pour into mixing bowl

Place fish into mixing bowl coating evenly (may use egg to help with coating)

Place fish onto baking sheet and drizzle with oil

Cooking

Place in oven at 375 F (200 C) for approximately 40 minutes until kumara chips are crispy

Look up cooking time of your preferred fish as cooking times vary, approximately 350 F (175 C) for 30 minutes

PALEO HAMBURGER

Hamburger Bun Ingredients

Dry

½ cup almond flour

¼ cup coconut flour

½ cup tapioca flour

1 tsp sea salt

1 tsp baking powder

Wet

½ cup applesauce

2 eggs

1 tbsp coconut oil

Paleo Mayonnaise Ingredients

1 egg yolk

2 tsp apple cider vinegar

½ tsp mustard

½ cup olive oil

5 tbsp coconut oil melted

Patty Ingredients

½ lb ground beef / ¼ kg mince

Salt and pepper to taste

Hamburger Buns Preparation

Mix dry ingredients together

Add wet ingredients and mix

Grease 2 Pyrex 2-cup baking dishes

Fill both dishes with batter to the top then place on a cooking sheet

Bake for 15 minutes at 350 F (175 C) (may need longer time to bake), check with a toothpick and when it comes out clean, remove from oven

Allow buns to cool then slice chicken

Mayonnaise Preparation

Place ingredients into measuring cup (or coffee cup), oil last

Mix using a hand-held immersion blender. Touch the bottom of the cup, blend on low, and bring up speed slowly (only takes a few seconds).

Use right away; will keep in refrigerator for a few days

Patty Preparation

Add spices to mince

Form 2 patties to desired size

Pan-fry in own juices.

Hamburger Preparation

Slice buns

Toast buns if desired

Spread thin layer of mayonnaise onto buns

Place patties onto buns

Add desired toppings to patties

(Courtesy of Mary Bamlet)

PALEO CHOCOLATE CHIP COOKIE BALLS

DRY INGREDIENTS

3 cups almond flour

4 tbsp coconut flour

1/2 tsp pink, Himalayan salt

2 cups mini chocolate chips (dairy, soy, and sugar-free)

WET INGREDIENTS

1 tbsp vanilla

1/3 cup raw honey

8 tbsp coconut oil

PREPARATION

Mix dry ingredients together

Add wet ingredients and mix

Place in refrigerator for 5 minutes so you can shape the dough into balls

1 rounded tbsp per ball

Chill for 20 minutes

(Courtesy of Mary Bamlet)

Made in the USA
Monee, IL
04 November 2026

67379720R00059